THE
LITTLE
Vitamin
AND
Mineral
ENCYCLOPEDIA

THE
LITTLE
Vitamin
AND
Mineral
ENCYCLOPEDIA

The Handbook of Vitamins and Minerals
for a Healthier Life

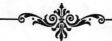

by Jack Ritchason

ISBN 0-86588-019-0

While every effort is made to guarantee the timeliness and authenticity of all information researched and presented in this publication, the ever-changing nature of the many activities underlying the facts, figures, trends, and theories presented makes impossible unqualified reliance on the material herein. Further, nothing herein is to be construed as a substitute for consultation with a qualified expert. Reasonable caution is the watchword of good health.

CONTENTS

About the Author

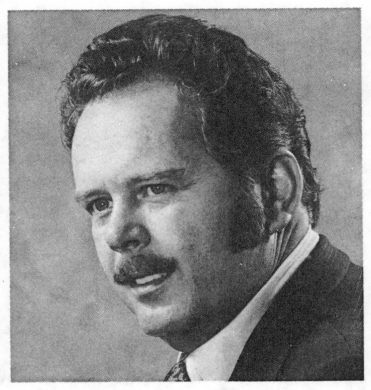

Dr. John (Jack) Ritchason

Dr. John (Jack) Ritchason has been in the health field for 17 years and has lectured nationally and internationally on herbs, vitamins, nutrition, and iridology. He graduated as a Naturopathic Doctor from Arizona College of Naturopathic Medicine, a branch of American University of Natural Therapeutics and Preventive Medicine. He is also a Registered Healthologist, Iridologist, Touch for Health Instructor, and Herbalist. He is a National Manager for Nature's Sunshine and is working on his Ph.D from Donsbach University.

INTRODUCTION

Life was intended to be rich and rewarding. Man was created and placed on earth to experience the full spectrum of life's opportunities. We have the capacity to know and enjoy the beauties of the natural world, the warmth of good interpersonal relationships, the fulfillment of achieving our goals. But central to our ability to enjoy life is the necessity of maintaining good health. The Apostle Paul understood this principle and wrote it to John: ". . . I wish above all things that thou mayest prosper and *be in health*. . ." (3 John:2).

All the Old Testament prophets were commanded to fast and to care for their bodies by making use of those natural foods available to them. Christ himself referred to his body as a temple (see John 2:21) and followed the pattern of fasting and using wholesome foods to maintain that temple.

The same principles are true for modern man: WE MUST SUSTAIN OURSELVES PHYSICALLY IN ORDER TO BE AT OUR BEST INTELLECTUALLY, SPIRITUALLY, AND EMOTIONALLY. The earth's abundance can still give us that sustenance, but our lives are now so complicated that we rarely can rely on diet alone to provide all the nutrients and chemicals our bodies require to function. Such commonplace and apparently harmless elements of daily living as refined sugars, white flour, city sunlight, daily stresses, cocktails, and aspirin actually rob us of the nutrients we need to live! It is no wonder that vitamin and mineral supplements are so vital to our health: they restore the natural substances our bodies use up in keeping us going.

EASY REFERENCE

The *Little Vitamin and Mineral Encyclopedia* puts the information you need about supplements right into your hands. You don't need to wade through pages of meaningless detail to find what you want. It includes alphabetical listings of conditions which respond to vitamin and mineral treatment and of the characteristics and uses of individual vitamins and minerals as well.

The information is basic, helpful, and easy to find. Simply bend the book vertically through the center; along the right edge you will see a handy thumb index to help you locate your desired subject quickly. The first section lists many common conditions which may be treated with vitamins and minerals. Several suggestions are made for each condition: you may find that one vitamin or one combination works better than another for you.

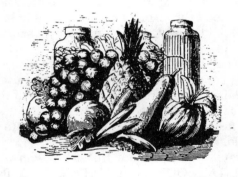

The second and third sections catalogue the vitamins and minerals themselves in alphabetical order, giving a little information about each one, listing the benefits of its use, and suggesting its best natural sources. It is intended that you may use these sections as a cross-reference with the first if you wish. In the paragraphs explaining benefits you will find key words in italics to draw your attention immediately to the ailments or conditions concerned. This makes it easier and faster for you to find a complete list of optional answers to your particular question.

For example, a quick glance at Section One will tell you vitamins C, K, and P might be helpful if you bruise easily. If you are interested in exactly how vitamin C affects bruises, simply look up vitamin C in Section Two and scan the page quickly until the word *bruises* catches your eye. Then you can immediately read exactly what you want to know about vitamin C without spending time looking through its other uses.

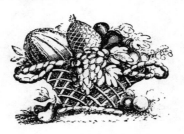

AILMENTS

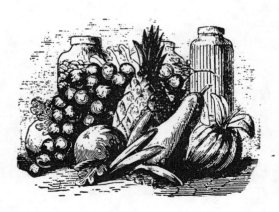

Vitamins and minerals generally work to support and encourage the body's natural functions. Deficiencies of vitamins and minerals can cause those functions to slow down, to occur inappropriately, or to fail. For this reason, deficiencies must be corrected.

Even those whose diets would supply all the vitamins and minerals they could normally use may have deficiencies for one reason or another. Stress at work, air pollution, pain, illness, even use of prescription drugs to combat disease can deplete vitamin and mineral supplies to deficiency levels. For this reason, regular supplements and a ready reference to symptoms and specific aids for problems as they arise can be your strongest ally in restoring and maintaining your health.

The beauty of vitamin and mineral treatment is that it is totally natural: it uses substances your body needs, substances your system was designed to use. Unlike treatment with drugs, vitamins and minerals add no foreign chemicals to the body, and they produce no side effects. They do not take control of the body; rather, they maintain an environment in which the body regains and sustains control of itself.

Of course, this does not mean that vitamin and mineral supplements can ward off or quickly cure serious illnesses. Vitamins and minerals help the body correct health problems. They do not correct inherited or chronic disorders or reverse the effects of critical health problems. The body is the master; vitamins and minerals are the tools and materials for the body to rebuild itself.

VITAMINS AND MINERALS DURING PREGNANCY

The old saying "You're eating for two now" is pretty widely acknowledged as false. While a pregnant woman does not eat for two, her body does supply nutrients to her unborn child, providing it with the material to develop normally. The expectant mother's energy requirements may increase as much as 300 calories per day; a nursing mother can expend an extra 1,000 calories a day. Obviously, these are conditions under which the health of both mother and baby are dependent upon the mother's understanding of her increased need for nutrients. The pregnant or nursing woman should supply herself a good multiple vitamin and mineral supplement and be particularly aware of getting enough vitamins B, C, and D and sufficient calcium and iron.

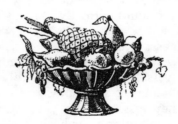

CHILDREN

Since vitamins and minerals effect the chemical reaction that changes food into useable proteins, carbohydrates and fats to build tissue and to supply energy, growing children need extra vitamins and minerals. They particularly require calcium and iron and B complex and C vitamins. Because kids expend so much energy and because they tend to supplement their diets themselves with sweets and junk foods, most of them get substantially fewer vitamins and minerals than they really need.

NOT PRESCRIPTIONS

The Little Vitamin and Mineral Encyclopedia does not directly or indirectly dispense medical advice or prescribe

ACNE

vitamin A, vitamin B_2, vitamin B_3, B complex, vitamin E, vitamin F, potassium, sulfur

ADRENAL GLAND

vitamin B_5, B complex

AGING

vitamin A, vitamin B_{13}, vitamin B_{15}, B complex, vitamin C, vitamin E, calcium, selenium

ALCOHOLISM

B complex, particularly vitamin B_1; vitamin B_{15}; folic acid; choline; potassium; zinc

ALLERGIES

B complex, particularly vitamin B_5; vitamin C; vitamin F; vitamin H; manganese; potassium

AMNESIA

vitamin B_6, vitamin B_{15}, B complex

ANEMIA

B complex, particularly vitamin B_1, vitamin B_6, and vitamin B_{12}; folic acid; vitamin C; vitamin E; vitamin T; cobalt; copper; iron; molybdenum

ANGINA

vitamin B_{15}, B complex, vitamin E

APPETITE

vitamin B1, vitamin B3, vitamin B12, B complex, folic acid, vitamin C, vitamin H, zinc

ARTERIOSCLEROSIS

vitamin A, vitamin B3, B complex, choline, vitamin D, vitamin E, chromium, zinc

ARTHRITIS

B complex, particularly vitamin B5; vitamin C; vitamin E; vitamin F; calcium; phosphorus; sulfur

ASTHMA

vitamin B12, vitamin B15, B complex, vitamin E

ATHEROSCLEROSIS

vitamin B6, vitamin B15, B complex, folic acid, choline, inositol, vitamin F, vitamin H, iodine, zinc

BAD BREATH

vitamin B3, vitamin B6, B complex

BALDNESS

B complex particularly vitamin B3, vitamin B5, vitamin B6, folic acid, and inositol; vitamin F; vitamin H; PABA; copper

BEE STINGS

vitamin B1, B complex, as repellant

BERIBERI

vitamin B_1, B complex

BIRTH DEFECTS

B complex, vitamin E, vitamin B_2 deficiency in mother may cause

BLINDNESS

B complex, vitamin A, vitamin B_2 (twilight blindness)

BLOOD

to build—B complex, vitamin B_5, vitamin B_6, folic acid, vitamin B_{12}, vitamin C, vitamin D, cobalt, iron; to encourage clotting—vitamin K; to encourage coagulation—vitamin T; to dissolve blood clots—vitamin E

BLOOD PRESSURE

to regulate—choline; to reduce high blood pressure—vitamin B_3, vitamin B_6, vitamin B_{15}, B complex, vitamin E, chromium, potassium

BOILS

vitamin A, vitamin C

BONES

vitamin A, vitamin C, vitamin D, calcium, fluorine, manganese, phosphorus

BONES (FRACTURED)

vitamin A, vitamin C, vitamin E, calcium

BRAIN

inositol, potassium, sulfur, zinc, lecithin

BRONCHITIS

vitamin A, vitamin C, vitamin E

BRUISES

vitamin C, vitamin K, vitamin P, calcium

BURNS

B complex, vitamin C, vitamin E, PABA, zinc

CANCER

vitamin B_{12}, vitamin B_{17}, B complex, vitamin C, selenium

CANKER SORES

vitamin B_3, B complex, folic acid

CARBUNCLES

vitamin A, vitamin C

CHICKEN POX

vitamin C, vitamin E, vitamin A

CHOLESTEROL

vitamin B_3, vitamin B_6, vitamin B_{15}, B complex, choline, vitamin F, inositol, vitamin C, lecithin, vanadium, zinc

CIRCULATORY SYSTEM

vitamin B_3, vitamin B_{15}, B complex, vitamin E, calcium, magnesium, niacin

COLDS

vitamin A, vitamin C, vitamin D, vitamin P, water

COLD SORES

vitamin A, vitamin C, vitamin E

COLITIS

vitamin B_6, B complex, vitamin E, vitamin K, calcium, iron

CONSTIPATION

choline, vitamin C, vitamin E, calcium, water

CONVULSIONS

vitamin B_6, B complex

CUTS

vitamin B_5, B complex, vitamin C, vitamin E, calcium

DANDRUFF

selenium

DEPRESSION

vitamin B_{12}, B complex, vitamin H, magnesium

DIABETES

B complex, vitamin E, chromium, manganese, potassium, zinc

DIARRHEA

vitamin B_1, vitamin B_3, B complex, folic acid

DIGESTION

for digestive problems—vitamin B_3, inositol, chlorine, magnesium, manganese; for converting foods into energy—vitamin B_1, vitamin B_2, vitamin B_5, vitamin B_6, vitamin B_{12}, B complex, folic acid, sodium

DIZZINESS

vitamin B_6, vitamin B_{15}, B complex, vitamin E, choline, vitamin P

DRY SKIN

vitamin A, vitamin D, vitamin E, vitamin F

EAR INFECTIONS

vitamin A, vitamin B_6, B complex, vitamin C, vitamin P

ECZEMA

vitamin A, B complex, inositol, vitamin F, vitamin H, PABA

EMPHYSEMA

vitamin A, vitamin B15, B complex, vitamin C, vitamin E, calcium

EXHAUSTION

vitamin B5, vitamin B12, vitamin B15, B complex, folic acid, vitamin C, vitamin D, vitamin E, vitamin H, iron, manganese, zinc

EYE DISORDERS

vitamin A, vitamin B2, vitamin B12, B complex, vitamin C, inositol, vitamin D, vitamin E, calcium

FATIGUE

vitamin B5, vitamin B15, B complex, vitamin C, vitamin E, vitamin H, iron, manganese

FOOT PROBLEMS

for discomfort—vitamin B1; for cold feet—take iodine; for athlete's foot—B complex, apply vitamin C powder

FEVER

vitamin A, vitamin B1, B complex, vitamin C, sodium, water

FOOD POISONING

folic acid

GANGRENE

vitamin B15, B complex, vitamin C, vitamin E

GASTROINTESTINAL SYSTEM

vitamin A, vitamin B3, B complex

GALLSTONES

vitamin A, vitamin B6, B complex, vitamin E, magnesium

GENITOURINARY SYSTEM

vitamin A, B complex, vitamin C, vitamin E

GLANDS

vitamin A, vitamin C

GOITER

iodine

GROWTH

vitamin B1, vitamin B2, vitamin B12, B complex, chromium, iodine, iron, phosphorus, zinc

GUMS

vitamin A, vitamin C, vitamin P, phosphorus

HAIR

vitamin A, vitamin B_2, vitamin B_6, B complex, folic acid, inositol, vitamin F, vitamin H, PABA, chlorine, iodine, sulfur

HANDS

for numbness—vitamin B_6; for cold hands—vitamin B_{15}, B complex, vitamin E, iodine

HANGOVERS

vitamin B_{15}, B complex

HAY FEVER

B complex, pantothenic acid, vitamin C

HEADACHE

B complex, particularly vitamin B_3, vitamin B_{15}, and choline; calcium and magnesium (ratio 2 to 1)

HEART

vitamin B_1, vitamin B_{15}, B complex, inositol, choline, vitamin D, vitamin E, vitamin F, vitamin K, calcium, magnesium, phosphorus, potassium, vanadium

HEMOPHILIA

vitamin T

HEMORRHOIDS

vitamin C, vitamin P

HERPES

vitamin A, vitamin B1, B complex, vitamin C

HYPERTHYROIDISM

vitamin A, vitamin B1, B complex, vitamin E, PABA, calcium

HYPOGLYCEMIA

vitamin B5, B complex, vitamin C, vitamin E, calcium

HYPOTHYROIDISM

iodine

IMPETIGO

vitamin A, vitamin C, vitamin E

INFECTIONS (RESISTING AND SPEEDING RECOVERY FROM)

vitamin A, vitamin B5, vitamin B15, B complex, vitamin C, vitamin P, iron, sulfur, water

INFERTILITY

vitamin E, zinc

INSOMNIA

vitamin B6, vitamin B15, B complex, folic acid, choline, calcium, iron

INTERNAL BLEEDING

vitamin C, vitamin K

INTESTINES

folic acid, inositol

IRRITABILITY

vitamin B_{12}, B complex, calcium, manganese

JOINTS

vitamin C, sulfur

KIDNEYS

vitamin B_6, B complex, choline, vitamin C, phosphorus

KIDNEY STONES

vitamin B_6, B complex, magnesium

LACTATION

vitamin B_1, vitamin B_2, B complex, folic acid, vitamin D

LEGS (CRAMPS)

vitamin B_1, vitamin B_3, vitamin B_6, vitamin B_{15}, B complex, vitamin E, vitamin H, calcium

LIPS

vitamin B_2, B complex

LIVER

vitamin A, vitamin B_1, vitamin B_6, vitamin B_{13}, vitamin B_{15}, B complex, insositol, choline, vitamin K, sulfur

LUNGS

vitamin A, vitamin E

MEASLES

vitamin A, vitamin C, vitamin E

MENOPAUSE

B complex, vitamin E, calcium, selenium

MENSTRUATION

B complex, particularly vitamin B_6; vitamin K; vitamin E; calcium; iron; zinc

MENTAL ATTITUDE

vitamin B_1, B complex, iodine

MENTAL CAPACITIES

vitamin B_{12}, B complex, choline, iodine, lecithin, manganese, potassium, zinc

MENTAL DISORIENTATION

vitamin B_3, vitamin B_{15}, B complex, calcium

MENTAL ILLNESS

vitamin B3, vitamin B12, folic acid, vitamin H, magnesium

MENTAL RETARDATION

vitamin B6, vitamin B15, B complex, vitamin D, vitamin E

METABOLISM

vitamin B1, vitamin B2, vitamin B5, vitamin B6, vitamin B12, B complex, folic acid, vitamin D, vitamin H, manganese, sodium

MIGRAINE HEADACHES

B complex, particularly vitamin B3

MISCARRIAGE (PREVENTION)

vitamin C, vitamin E, vitamin P

MONONUCLEOSIS

vitamin A, B complex, vitamin C, potassium

MORNING SICKNESS

vitamin B1, vitamin B6, B complex, vitamin K

MOTION SICKNESS

vitamin B1, vitamin B6, B complex

MOUTH

vitamin B2, vitamin B3, vitamin B5, vitamin B6, B complex

MUCOUS MEMBRANES

vitamin A, vitamin B2, B complex

MULTIPLE SCLEROSIS

vitamin B13, B complex, lecithin, vitamin E

MUSCLES

vitamin B1, vitamin B6, B complex, choline, vitamin C, vitamin E, vitamin H, calcium, magnesium, manganese, sodium

MUSCULAR DYSTROPHY

inositol, vitamin E, B complex, calcium

NAILS

vitamin A, vitamin B2, B complex, iodine, sulfur, zinc

NEPHRITIS

vitamin B6, B complex, vitamin C, vitamin E

NERVOUS SYSTEM

vitamin A, vitamin B1, vitamin B3, vitamin B6, vitamin B12, B complex, choline, vitamin E, calcium, magnesium, manganese, sodium

NEURITIS

vitamin B1, B complex

NIGHT BLINDNESS

vitamin A

NOSEBLEEDS

vitamin C, vitamin K, calcium

NURSING

vitamin B_1, vitamin B_2, B complex, folic acid, vitamin D

OSTEOMALACIA

vitamin D, calcium

OVERWEIGHT

B complex, particularly vitamin B_6; inositol, choline; vitamin F; calcium; iodine; magnesium

PALSY

vitamin B_6, B complex, vitamin E

PAIN

vitamin B_1, B complex; folic acid; vitamin K; calcium; vitamin C for back, neck, and leg pain due to injury of spinal disc

PELLAGRA

vitamin B_3, vitamin B_6

PHLEBITIS

vitamin C, vitamin E, lecithin

POISON IVY

vitamin A, vitamin C, vitamin E

PROSTATE DISORDERS

vitamin E, vitamin F, zinc

PSORIASIS

vitamin A, inositol, vitamin C, vitamin E

REPRODUCTIVE SYSTEM

vitamin A, vitamin B2, B complex, vitamin E, manganese

RESPIRATORY SYSTEM

vitamin A, vitamin E

RESTLESSNESS

vitamin B3, vitamin B6, B complex, calcium

RHEUMATIC FEVER

vitamin A, B complex, vitamin C, vitamin E, vitamin P, PABA

RHEUMATISM

vitamin B15, B complex, vitamin F, vitamin P, calcium

RICKETS

vitamin D, calcium, phosphorus

SCURVY

vitamin A, vitamin B_1, vitamin B_3, B complex, vitamin C

SHINGLES

vitamin B_{12}, B complex, calcium

SHOCK

vitamin B_5, B complex, vitamin C

SINUSITIS

vitamin A, vitamin B_5, B complex, vitamin C, vitamin E

SKIN

vitamin A, vitamin B_2, vitamin B_3, vitamin B_6, B complex, vitamin D, vitamin E, folic acid, vitamin F, vitamin H, PABA, iodine, iron, sulfur

SKIN DISORDERS

vitamin A, vitamin B_3, vitamin B_5, vitamin B_6, vitamin B_{12}, B complex, vitamin D, inositol, vitamin E, vitamin F, vitamin H, PABA, sulfur (in creams)

SNAKEBITE

vitamin A, vitamin C, vitamin K

SORES

vitamin A, vitamin B2, vitamin B3, B complex, vitamin C, vitamin E, folic acid

SORE THROAT

vitamin A, vitamin B2, vitamin C, iodine

SPINAL DISC

vitamin C, calcium, sulfur

STRESS (MENTAL AND PHYSICAL)

B complex, particularly vitamin B2, vitamin B5, vitamin B6, vitamin B15, folic acid, vitamin C, vitamin E, PABA, magnesium, phosphorus

SUNBURN

B complex, vitamin C, PABA

SUNSTROKE

B complex, vitamin C, sodium

TASTE

zinc

TEETH

vitamin A, vitamin B3, vitamin B5, vitamin B6, B complex, vitamin C, vitamin D, calcium, chlorine, fluorine, iodine, magnesium, phosphorus

THROMBOSIS

vitamin E

TONGUE

vitamin B2, vitamin B3, B complex

ULCERS

vitamin A, B complex, folic acid, vitamin C, vitamin E, vitamin P, vitamin U, calcium

VARICOSE VEINS

vitamin C, vitamin E, calcium

VENEREAL DISEASE

vitamin A, vitamin C, and vitamin K to replenish after antiboiotics

VISION

vitamin A, vitamin B2, vitamin B3, B complex, vitamin C, vitamin E

WARTS

vitamin A, vitamin E

WEAKNESS

vitamin B1, vitamin B6, B complex, vitamin C, vitamin E

WEIGHT LOSS

vitamin B1, vitamin B6, B complex

WOUNDS

vitamin A, vitamin B5, B complex, vitamin C, vitamin E, zinc

VITAMINS

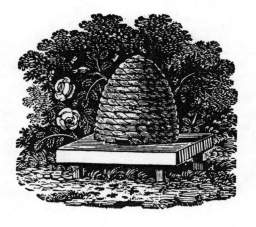

Vitamins are organic substances necessary for life. We have to ingest vitamins in or with our food. As a matter of fact, the body cannot use vitamins without minerals.

The food we eat is composed of proteins, carbohydrates, and fats which the body converts into energy in a form it can use. In order to do that, the body must have the proper amounts and kinds of vitamins. Balanced vitamins act like a catalyst for use of other nutrients: they are not themselves used, but they start and maintain the chemical reaction through which you burn calories and use up the fuel that feeds your body.

Most vitamins are water soluble. That is, they combine with water in the body to do their job, and then they are carried off and excreted in the urine. Most vitamins remain in your system for two-to-three hours at the longest before they are eliminated. In order to assure day-long vitamin levels, water-soluble vitamins must be taken regularly—either by eating a proper diet or by taking supplemental vitamins such as found in tablet or capsule form. The oil-soluble vitamins—A, D, and E—need for fat assimilation. If for some reason your diet does not include sufficient fat, the oil-soluble vitamins are available in "dry" or water-soluble form.

In any case, vitamins should be taken before—not between and not in place of—meals. Ideally, they should be taken with breakfast, with lunch, and with dinner, but if your schedule allows you only one time a day for vitamins, make that time with breakfast and try to use time release vitamins. Feed your body every five hours for maximum efficiency.

Try to balance your vitamins to work together. The B complex, for example, is a group of twenty-two similar vitamins. Even though they are all distinct, none of them works as well alone as the entire group does together. They are never found singly in nature; they are always all there. Other vitamins have partners as well; it is a good idea to combine them for effectiveness.

Vitamin A functions best with—B complex, vitamin D, vitamin E, calcium, phosphorus, and zinc.

Vitamin D functions best with—vitamin A, vitamin C, choline, calcium, and phosphorus.

Vitamin E functions best with—B complex, inositol, vitamin C, and manganese.

Vitamin C (ascorbic acid) functions best with—bioflavonoids, calcium, and magnesium.

Folic acid (folacin) functions best with—B complex and vitamin C.

Niacin functions best with—vitamin B_1, vitamin B_2, B complex, and vitamin C.

Vitamin B_1 (thiamine) functions best with—B complex, B_2, folic acid, niacin, vitamin C, and vitamin E.

Vitamin B_2 (riboflavin) functions best with—vitamin B_6, B complex, vitamin C, and niacin.

Vitamin B_6 (pyridoxine) functions best with—vitamin B_1, vitamin B_2, B complex, pantothenic acid, vitamin C, and magnesium.

Vitamin B_{12} (cyanocobalamin) functions best with—vitamin B_6, B complex, vitamin C, folic acid, choline, inositol, and potassium.

Calcium functions best with—vitamin A, vitamin C, vitamin D, iron, magnesium, and phosphorus.

Phosphorus functions best with—calcium, vitamin A, vitamin D, iron, and manganese.

Iron functions best with—vitamin B_{12}, folic acid, vitamin C, and calcium.

Magnesium functions best with—vitamin B6, vitamin C, vitamin D, calcium, and phosphorus.

Zinc functions best with—vitamin A, calcium, and phosphorus.

A few vitamins may have toxic effects if taken in massive doses over a long period of time. Watch intake of vitamins A and D; avoid combining vitamin A with mineral oil or vitamin E with inorganic iron. It is typically synthetic vitamins which cause reactions. Natural vitamins, even in high doses, are safe.

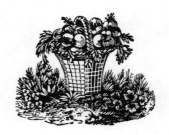

VITAMIN A

Because vitamin A is fat soluble, it requires fats as well as minerals for proper absorption in the digestive tract.

The body can store vitamin A, so daily intake is not necessary. As a matter of fact, large daily doses of vitamin A over a period of months can produce toxic effects. The average dosage of vitamin A is 25,000 to 100,000 units depending on body stresses.

Benefits

In general, vitamin A serves to maintain the body's thin coverings and also its mucous membranes in various organs, systems, and glands. Specifically, vitamin A:

- counteracts *night blindness* and helps heal various disorders of the *eyes* and *vision*

- helps treat such *skin problems* as acne, impetigo, psoriasis, boils, carbuncles, and open ulcers when applied directly

- builds resistance to *colds* and to *infections*, particularly in the *gastrointestinal*, *urinary*, and respiratory systems

- promotes healing of *broken bones* and *damaged skin or organs*

- maintains healthy functioning of the *liver* and *reproductive organs*

- aids in treatment of *emphysema* and *hyperthyroidism*

- promotes *growth* and *maintenance* of healthy *bones*, *skin*, *hair*, *teeth* and *gums*

- maintains *balance* of *sex hormones*

- shortens the duration of *diseases*

Natural sources

Green and yellow vegetables, eggs, milk and dairy products, margarine, yellow fruits, liver, fish liver oil, lemon grass.

VITAMIN B1 (THIAMINE)

Vitamin B1 is necessary for the body to make full use of its carbohydrate intake.

Sometimes called the "morale vitamin," B1 strengthens the nervous system and can improve mental attitude. It helps all kinds of stress, so the need for this vitamin increases during illness, trauma, anxiety, and postsurgical periods.

Women who are pregnant, nursing, or taking birth control pills have increased needs for vitamin B1, as do smokers, drinkers, and those who consume a great deal of sugar or caffeine.

Vitamin B1 is water soluble and must be replaced daily.

Benefits

- necessary in treatment of *beriberi, neuritis,* and *alcoholism*
- *aids digestion,* particularly of carbohydrates
- helps fight *air-* or *seasickness*
- *maintains* normal functioning of the *nervous system, muscles, heart*
- aids in *treatment* of herpes zoster
- helps relieve *dental postoperative pain*
- promotes *growth*
- improves *mental attitude*
- repels *biting insects*

Natural sources:

Whole wheat, oatmeal, peanuts, bran, most vegetables, milk, rice husks, dried yeast.

VITAMIN B2 (RIBOFLAVIN)

Vitamin B2 helps the body digest fats, proteins, and carbohydrates and convert them into energy it can use.

Those who may be deficient in this vitamin include people who habitually skip meals, refuse to eat liver or green vegetables, or follow a restrictive diet (as for ulcers, colitis, or diabletes) over a long period of time. Alcoholism may also lead to B2 deficiency.

Vitamin B2 must be replaced daily.

Benefits

- helps clear up *lesions* of the *mouth, lips, skin, genitalia*

- benefits *vision*, alleviates *eye fatigue*, prevents *twilight blindness*

- helps eliminate *sore mouth, lips, tongue*

- promotes healthy *skin, nails, hair*

- aids in *growth and reproduction*

- functions with other substances to *metabolize* carbohydrates, fats, proteins

- aids in *stress* situations

Natural sources

Liver, kidney, fish, eggs, cheese, milk, yeast, leafy green vegetables.

VITAMIN B3 (NIACIN)

Vitamin B3 is necessary for a healthy nervous system and proper brain function. A lack of this vitamin can cause negative personality changes.

Vitamin B3 is also essential for the body to produce cortisone, thyroxine, insulin, and male and female sex hormones.

The body can usually produce its own vitamin B3, but only if it is receiving enough vitamins B1, B2, and B6.

If you are taking extra vitamin B3, you may notice a flushing and itching of the skin—this is normal and should not last long.

Vitamin B3 must be replaced daily.

Benefits

- combats *pellagra, confusion, digestive difficulties,* and *blotched skin;* relieves such symptoms as *perceptual changes* ("hearing things" or "seeing things" that aren't there).

- counteracts arteriosclerosis (hardening of the arteries)

- *reduces cholesterol*

- increases circulation and reduces high blood pressure

- helps prevent or make less severe migraine headaches

- promotes a *healthy digestive system* and *alleviates digestive problems*

- eliminates canker sores and improves *skin's general appearance*

- *eases* some attacks of diarrhea

- sometimes *helps eliminate bad breath*

Natural sources

Liver, lean meat, kidney, fish, eggs, the white meat of poultry, whole wheat, yeast, wheat germ, roasted peanuts, avocados, dates, figs, prunes.

VITAMIN B5 (PANTOTHENIC ACID)

Vitamin B5 is necessary in the production of various hormones.

It is also used to build antibodies and to convert foods into useable energy.

It helps in the production of new cells and the maintenance of normal growth and resistance to stress.

Benefits

- helps control *hypoglycemia*
- aids in preventing *duodenal ulcers*
- fights *infections* and *disease*
- prevents *fatigue*
- aids in healing *wounds*
- speeds recovery after *surgery*
- reduces *negative effects of antibiotics*
- helps prevent *blood and skin disorders*
- eases pain of *arthritis*

Natural sources

Meats, kidney, heart, liver, chicken, nuts, whole grains, wheat germ, bran, yeast, molasses, green vegetables, tomatoes, potatoes.

VITAMIN B6 (PYRIDOXINE)

Vitamin B6 is primarily useful in assuring proper chemical balance in the blood and body tissues. It is essential in helping the body produce niacin (vitamin B3), so a shortage of B6 may be indicated by the symptoms of B3 deficiency.

It also helps the body convert fats and proteins into useful energy, and it helps maintain salt and water balances.

Vitamin B6 is necessary for the production of antibodies and red blood cells.

Those whose diets are high in protein and women who take birth control pills are likely to need extra vitamin B6.

Vitamin B6 must be replaced daily.

Benefits

- helps treat *anemia*
- *alleviates nausea*, specifically *morning sickness*
- controls *cholesterol* level in blood
- reduces *muscle spasms*, particularly cramps and numbness which occur at night
- promotes healthy *skin, teeth, muscles,* and *nerves*
- helps prevent *kidney and gallstones*
- builds resistance to *ear infections*
- eases *air-* and *seasickness*

Natural sources

Lean meats, liver, kidney, heart, milk, eggs, soybeans, nuts, yeast, wheat bran, wheat germ, cantaloupe, bananas, molasses, and leafy green vegetables.

VITAMIN B12 (COBALAMIN)

Vegetarians risk deficiency in vitamin B12 and so should supplement their diets with this vitamin. Women who are pregnant or nursing also benefit from additional B12.

Because it is sometimes difficult for the body to absorb B12, it should be combined with calcium.

Vitamin B12 is effective in very small doses.

Benefits

- prevents *anemia*
- helps ease *asthma*
- promotes *growth* and increases *appetite* in children
- prevents *eye damage*, particularly from smoke or pollution
- increases *energy*
- relieves *irritability*
- maintains *nervous system*
- aids *digestion*
- helps improve *concentration, memory,* and *balance*

Natural sources

Liver, kidney, beef, saltwater fish, oysters, eggs, milk, cheese.

VITAMIN B13 (OROTIC ACID)

Very little research has yet been done on vitamin B13.

It is not currently available in the United States, but it can be obtained in Europe.

Benefits

- possibly prevents some *liver problems*
- aids in treatment of *multiple sclerosis*
- helps prevent *premature aging*

Natural sources

Root vegetables (carrots, potatoes, turnips, etc.), whey, liquid from curdled milk.

VITAMIN B15 (PANGAMIC ACID)

The essential requirement for vitamin B15 has not been proved. It is enthusiastically used in Russia, but the U.S. Food and Drug Administration has given some resistance to its sale in the United States.

Some people become slightly nauseated for a little while after starting to take B15, but this usually lasts only a few days. Taking the vitamin after the day's largest meal helps ease this nausea.

B15 acts more effectively if taken together with vitamins A and E.

Russians recommend taking 50 mg three times a day for 90 days, cutting back then to one a day.

Benefits

- stops the *craving for liquor*
- speeds recovery from *fatigue*
- protects against *pollutants*
- helps lower *cholesterol* level
- increases *immunity* to infections
- relieves symptoms of *angina* and *asthma*
- helps prevent *cirrhosis*
- aids in easing *hangovers*

Natural sources

Whole grains, whole brown rice, pumpkin seeds, sesame seeds, yeast.

VITAMIN B17 (LAETRILE)

Vitamin B17 is very controversial. It has been rejected by the U.S. Food and Drug Administration, and its use in cancer treatment is legal only in parts of the United States.

Massive doses of B17 should never be taken all at once. It is better to take small doses at different times during the day. It is recommended to take in addition to B17 large doses of vitamin A (in emulsion form) and large doses of enzymes.

Benefits

- may aid in preventing or controlling some *cancers*

Natural sources

The pits of apricots, cherries, peaches, plums, nectarines, apples.

VITAMIN B FACTORS (INOSITOL)

Inositol seems to be most effective when taken together with other vitamins, particularly vitamin E, choline, and biotin.

Inositol appears to be important in the proper function of the heart, eyes, and brain.

Benefits

- prevents *eczema*
- promotes healthy *hair* and helps prevent *hair loss*
- regulates *cholesterol levels* and aids in treatment of *atherosclerosis*
- aids in redistribution of *body fat*
- builds resistance to *cirrhosis of the liver*
- helps in treatment of *nerve damage* from some types of *muscular dystrophy*
- counteracts *negative effects of caffeine*

Natural sources

Organ meats (liver, heart, brains), peanuts, dried lima beans, yeast, molasses, wheat germ, raisins, cantaloupe, grapefruit, cabbage.

VITAMIN B FACTORS (CHOLINE)

Choline is necessary in liver development and in maintaining the functions of both liver and kidney.

It is also required in the thin covering of nerve fibers—a deficiency of choline can damage the nerves and so impair body functions.

Benefits

- helps control *cholesterol*
- sustains healthy *nerves, kidneys, liver*
- maintains *muscles*
- helps control *blood pressure*
- aids those nerve impulses that affect *memory*
- assists liver in *eliminating poisons* from the blood

Natural sources

Organ meats, egg yolks, yeast, wheat germ, peanuts or peanut butter, green leafy vegetables, various seeds.

VITAMIN B FACTORS (FOLIC ACID)

Folic acid is most effective when taken together with vitamin B12. In turn, it is necessary for the full effectiveness of vitamins A, D, E, and K.

Those who should increase their folic acid intake include people who take large doses of vitamin C, women who are pregnant (particularly just before delivery) or nursing, women who take birth control pills, and persons who drink alcoholic beverages.

Benefits

- helps prevent *anemia*
- improves *lactation*
- aids in reducing *pain*
- protects against *intestinal parasites and food poisoning*
- sometimes helps delay the *graying of hair* (when used with pantothenic acid and PABA)
- increases *appetite* in those who are run down
- promotes *healthy-looking skin*
- helps prevent *canker sores*

Natural sources

Liver, egg yolks, yeast, bran, avocados, pumpkins, cantaloupe, apricots, whole wheat, dark rye flour, deep-green leafy vegetables, carrots.

VITAMIN C (ASCORBIC ACID)

Vitamin C is essential for the body to produce collagen, which is the substance that bonds cells together. Maintaining vitamin C in your body therefore helps preserve and mend the connective tissues (tendons and cartilage—including the cartilage between spinal discs), bones, muscles, and blood vessels.

Vitamin C also helps the body use iron.

You need extra vitamin C if you:

—smoke

—take aspirin often

—live or work in a city or other environment with carbon monoxide in the air

—take birth control pills.

Vitamin C must be replaced daily.

Benefits

- prevents scurvy

- helps prevent or make less severe the common cold

- promotes healing of wounds, burns, and bone fractures

- increases resistance to infections, fatigue, and low temperatures

- aids in prevention of internal bleeding, from ulcers to simple bruises

- helps guard against anemia

- maintains solid bones and teeth

- promotes healthy gums

- helps relieve back problems and related discomforts

- acts as a mild diuretic

- helps body meet various stresses

- encourages healing after surgery

- aids in decreasing cholesterol level in the blood

- reduces discomforts of allergies

- gives a high resistance to *cancer*

Natural sources

Citrus fruits (oranges, grapefruit, lemons, limes, tomatoes), green leafy vegetables, broccoli, cauliflower, berries, cantaloupe, potatoes.

VITAMIN D

Vitamin D is necessary for the body to build calcium in the bones. It is also required to release the calcium for the body's use. Because of this, vitamin D deficiency is usually related to calcium deficiency conditions.

We can receive vitamin D directly from the sunshine as well as through diet. Those whose clothing, environment, or work schedules limit their exposure to the sun should probably increase the vitamin D in their diets. It should be noted that once a suntan is established, the skin no longer absorbs vitamin D from the sun.

Women who are pregnant or nursing need extra vitamin D, as do children who are still growing.

Benefits

- prevents *rickets*
- helps prevent *osteomalacia* and some *irregularities in heartbeat*
- builds strong *bones* and *teeth*
- aids in producing *blood plasma*
- is effective in treatment of *keratoconus (distention of the cornea)*
- relieves *chronic conjunctivitis*
- prevents *colds* when taken with vitamins A and C
- helps body use *calcium, phosphorus and vitamin A*

Natural sources

Milk, dairy products, ultraviolet sun rays, egg yolk, fish liver oils, sardines, herring, salmon, tuna.

VITAMIN E

Vitamin E acts to control the unsaturated fatty acids in the body; it affects virtually all body tissues.

Vitamin E is more potent when taken together with selenium.

Vitamin E boosts the action of vitamin A.

Those who drink chlorinated water and women who are pregnant, nursing, taking birth control pills, or going through the menopause may need extra vitamin E.

Vitamin E may be <u>applied directly in treatment of wounds or other skin disorders.</u>

Vitamin E is not retained in the body and should be replaced regularly.

Benefits

- strengthens and protects reproductive, muscular, circulatory, skeletal, and nervous systems

- improves circulation

- helps prevent arteriosclerosis and blood clots

- useful in treating gangrene, nephritis, rheumatic fever, purpura, retinitis, diabetes mellitus, congenital heart disease, phlebitis

- prevents or lessens scar tissue, both internal and external, and so is helpful after surgery or heart attack

- aids healing of wounds, burns, chronic ulcers, and some skin diseases

- protects respiratory system from pollution

- increases fertility

- prevents premature aging

- improves endurance

- acts as a mild diuretic (and may therefore lower blood pressure)

- helps prevent miscarriage

- counteracts *fatigue*
- strengthens *heart*
- carries *oxygen*
- goes straight to *placenta*

Natural sources

Wheat germ, vegetable oils, peanuts, whole-grain cereals, green leafy vegetables, broccoli, spinach, eggs.

VITAMIN F (UNSATURATED FATTY ACIDS)

The unsaturated fatty acids provide the body with fats in a form which can be used. They also aid in burning up the saturated fats already in the system.

Vitamin F is best absorbed if taken with vitamin E.

Those whose diets include a great deal of carbohydrates need additional vitamin F.

Benefits

- prevents *eczema* and *acne*
- aids in *weight reduction*
- helps control *cholesterol* levels
- encourages healthy *hair* and *skin*
- provides some protection against *negative effects of x-rays*

Natural sources

Oils of wheat germ, linseed, corn, cottonseed, sunflower, safflower, soybean, and peanut; walnuts, almonds, pecans, peanuts, avocados.

VITAMIN H (BIOTIN)

Vitamin H helps the liver produce lipids (fats) and promotes the conversion of food into energy.

Vitamin H is necessary to utilize vitamin C.

Raw egg whites counteract vitamin H, so those who eat or drink mixtures containing raw egg should increase their vitamin H.

Benefits

- helps prevent *eczema*
- eases *muscle pain*
- aids *metabolism*
- helps prevent baldness and graying of hair
- builds resistance to some *allergies*
- alleviates or prevents *exhaustion*

Natural sources

Green leafy vegetables, nuts, fruits, unrefined rice, egg yolks, liver, kidney, milk.

VITAMIN K

Besides its uses in the human body, vitamin K works as an excellent preservative for food. It does not alter the taste or appearance of the food it preserves.

Benefits

- helps prevent *colitis*
- promotes adequate *blood clotting*
- reduces susceptibility to *nose bleeds*
- works to counteract *nausea* in pregnant women
- reduces excessive *menstrual flow*
- prevents *internal hemorrhaging*
- aids in treating *snakebite*
- helps relieve *pain*

Natural sources

Yogurt, green leafy vegetables, root vegetables (carrots, potatoes, turnips), alfalfa, safflower oil, soybean oil, kelp.

VITAMIN P (BIOFLAVONOIDS)

Vitamin P is essential for the proper absorption and use of vitamin C. These two vitamins work together to strengthen capillaries and connective tissues.

When you buy *natural* vitamin C, you usually get vitamin P as well.

Benefits

- prevents *bruising*
- helps treat *edema* and <u>*dizziness*</u> which result from *inner ear* infections
- builds resistance to *infection*
- prevents *bleeding gums*
- helps prevent *miscarriage*
- eases and speeds recovery from *influenza* and the *common cold*
- helps counteract *hemorrhages* caused by *anticoagulant drugs.*
- boosts action of vitamin C

Natural sources

Citrus fruits (primarily the white skin and the segment membranes), apricots, blackberries, cherries, grapes, plums, rose hips.

PABA

PABA helps the body make folic acid and use pantothenic acid (vitamin B5).

It is destroyed by some antibiotics and sulfa drugs, so PABA intake should be increased while taking those medications.

Benefits

- helps prevent *eczema*
- aids in healing and relieving pain of burns
- keeps *skin* healthy and helps prevent *wrinkles*
- screens the sun and prevents *sunburn* when applied directly to the skin
- helps restore *natural hair color*

Natural sources

Organ meats (liver, kidney), yeast, whole grains, wheat germ, bran.

VITAMIN T

Very little research has been done for this vitamin.

Benefits

- helps *blood coagulation*
- prevents some kinds of *anemia* and *hemophilia*

Natural sources

Egg yolks, sesame seeds.

VITAMIN U

Little is known about this vitamin.

Benefits

- maybe helps heal *ulcers*

Natural sources

Raw cabbage.

MINERALS

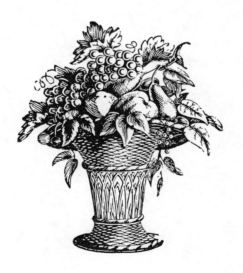

Minerals are necessary to regulate body functions and to maintain tissues. Minerals, as well as vitamins, must be supplied daily either in the diet or through supplements.

Minerals are necessary for the body to be able to use vitamins. Minerals are the spark plugs of vitamin use. You can see that this chain of digestive chemical reactions is complicated and interrelated. Without vitamins and minerals you could eat everything in sight and still be malnourished.

To complicate things further, minerals cannot be used by the body unless they have been broken down into a digestible form. This process is called chelation (pronounced *key'lation*), and it frequently costs you up to half the amount of mineral you take. Because of this, it is both cheaper and wiser to purchase mineral supplements in chelated form. Cutting this one step out of the work your body has to do to use the fuel you feed it makes a big difference in the effectiveness of the nutritional process.

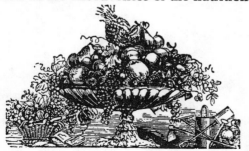

Research done in Poland has shown that vitamins and minerals put in a base of herbs will raise the body's ability to use those vitamins and minerals four-to-five times better than it would be able to without the herbs. This is a form of natural chelation; any vitamin and mineral product assembled this way is naturally chelated.

Vitamins are organic. That is, they are built of chemical structures based on carbon. But minerals are not basically carbons (with the exception of a few organic irons). Just the right combinations of vitamins and minerals are very important. Keep the following guidelines in mind as you plan your balanced diet.

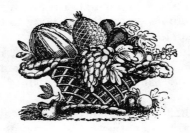

CALCIUM

Calcium and phosphorus should be balanced two-to-one in the human body.

Vitamin D is necessary for proper use of calcium.

Growing children and hypoglycemics benefit from increased calcium intake.

Calcium helps the body use iron.

Benefits

- prevents *rickets*
- promotes growth and maintenance of healthy *teeth and bones*
- maintains *cardiovascular system*, including regulating *heart beat*
- supports *nervous system*, particularly transmission of *nerve impulses;* calms nerves
- increases a person's ability to withstand pain
- relieves muscle spasms
- relieves *menstrual cramps*
- helps treat *insomnia*
- eases "*growing pains*"
- nothing heals without enough *calcium*

Natural sources

Milk and dairy products, cheese, peanuts, sunflower seeds, walnuts, soybeans, dried beans, green vegetables, salmon, sardines.

CHROMIUM

Benefits

- helps prevent *diabetes*
- deters *arteriosclerosis*
- aids *growth*
- helps prevent and correct *high blood pressure*

Natural sources

Meat, shellfish, clams, chicken, corn oil, yeast.

CHLORINE

Most people who eat an average amount of sea salt each day get adequate chlorine.

Those whose water is chlorinated should eat yogurt to restore intestinal bacteria. They should also increase their intake of vitamin C and vitamin E.

Benefits

- promotes healthy *teeth* and *hair*
- aids *digestion*

Natural sources

Sea salt, olives, kelp.

COBALT

Very strict vegetarians are likely to need supplementary cobalt.

Benefits

- helps prevent *anemia*
- builds *red blood cells*

Natural sources

Meat, kidney, liver, clams, oysters, milk.

COPPER

Most people who eat balanced diets get adequate copper. Supplementary copper is rarely prescribed and care should be taken not to over-treat oneself with it. Excessive amounts of copper can keep you awake at night, cause irregular menstrual periods, bring on depression, or increase hair loss.

Copper is required for the body to make proper use of iron and vitamin C.

Benefits

- maintain *high energy level*
- helps prevent *anemia* and *edema*

Natural sources

Whole wheat, dried beans, peas, liver, shrimp, most seafood, prunes.

FLUORINE

Synthetic fluorine is a toxic poison in water, vitamins, and toothpaste. Natural fluorine is beneficial to the body. An excess of either natural or synthetic fluorine can cause mottling or discoloration to the teeth. Fluorine is an essential trace mineral concentrated in the teeth and bones. It helps the body in the use of calcium.

Benefits

- strengthens *bones*
- builds resistance to *tooth decay*

Natural sources

Seafoods, gelatin, whole wheat, garlic, beets, lettuce, cabbage, radishes, egg whites.

IODINE

Sufficient iodine for most people is supplied in regular multivitamin and mineral tablets. Those who live in regions where the soil is iodine-poor (the Midwest, for example) and women who are pregnant or nursing might need more.

Benefits

- helps prevent *goiter* and *hypothyroidism*
- encourages *growth*
- boosts *energy level*
- helps system *burn excess fat*
- aids in maintaining *mental alertness* and the ability to *think quickly*
- promotes healthy *hair, skin, teeth,* and *nails*

Natural sources

Seafood, kelp, vegetables grown in rich soil.

IRON

Iron is necessary for the body to absorb and use B vitamins.

In turn, vitamin C and copper, cobalt, and manganese must be present for the body to use iron.

Those who should take extra iron include menstruating women and those who drink large amounts of coffee or tea.

Benefits

- prevents and helps treat *anemia*
- promotes *growth*
- builds *resistance to disease*
- restores healthy *skin tone*
- guards against *fatigue*

Natural sources

Red meat, organ meats (liver, kidney, heart), egg yolks, clams, oysters, dried peaches, nuts, beans, asparagus, oatmeal.

MAGNESIUM

Magnesium is essential for the body to be able to use calcium and vitamin C.

It helps convert blood sugar into usable energy.

Women who take birth control pills and anyone who drinks alcohol should increase their magnesium.

Since magnesium neutralizes stomach acids, it should not be taken directly after a meal.

Benefits

- helps prevent *heart attack* and keeps the *cardiovascular system* healthy

- relieves *indigestion*

- aids in resisting *depression*

- helps prevent *calcium deposits* and *kidney stones and gallstones*

- improves *dental health*

Natural sources

Yellow corn, dark green vegetables, lemons, grapefruit, figs, nuts, seeds, apples.

MANGANESE

Those who drink a great deal of milk or eat a large amount of meat may need additional manganese.

Benefits

- promotes proper *development and function* of central *nervous system, thyroid hormones,* and *skeletal and reproductive systems*
- required in *digestion* and *metabolism* of food
- improves *reflexes*
- reduces *irritability*
- eliminates *fatigue*
- improves *memory*

Natural sources

Whole-grain cereals, nuts, peas, green leafy vegetables, beets, egg yolks.

MOLYBDENUM

Molybdenum helps the body convert food into usable energy. It also contributes to the utilization of iron.

Most people get adequate molybdenum in their diets.

Benefits

- helps prevent *anemia*

Natural sources

Dark green leafy vegetables, peas, beans, nuts, whole grains.

PHOSPHORUS

Phosphorus requires calcium (ratio 1-to-2) in order to work. Vitamin D is also necessary for phosphorus to be effective.

Benefits

- prevents *rickets* and *pyorrhea*
- builds healthy *bones and teeth*
- aids regular *heartbeat* and normal *kidney function*
- decreases *arthritis* pain
- promotes general *growth* and *healing* of tissues

Natural sources

Fish, poultry, meat, eggs, seeds, nuts, whole grains.

POTASSIUM

Conditions which may indicate need for additional potassium include hypoglycemia, severe diarrhea, mental or physical stress, long periods of fasting or dieting. The increase of the use of salt as a preservative has increased the need for potassium.

Benefits

- helps keep *heart rhythms* normal
- aids in regulating body's *water balance*
- encourages *clear thinking*
- helps control *allergies*
- aids in disposal of *body wastes*
- helps reduce *blood pressure*

Natural sources

Citrus fruits, green leafy vegetables, watercress, mint leaves, sunflower seeds, bananas, potatoes.

SELENIUM

Selenium works best in combination with vitamin E.

In general, men need a little more selenium than women do.

Benefits

- slows down *aging* process
- prevents *heart* disease
- maintains *elasticity* in tissues
- helps treat and prevent *dandruff*
- may provide protection from certain *cancers*
- combats *harmful metals* in our environment

Natural sources

Bran, wheat germ, tuna, tomatoes, onions, broccoli.

SODIUM

Most people eat much more salt than they realize or than they need to eat. It is easier to add sodium to your diet than to eliminate or cut down on it.

An excess of sodium may contribute to high blood pressure.

It is recommended that most people cut their salt intake. However, for those *few* who need extra salt, kelp is an ideal supplement.

Benefits

- prevents *sunstroke* and *heat prostration*
- aids in proper function of *muscles* and *nerves*
- promotes *digestion of carbohydrates*
- in some cases helps prevent *neuralgia*

Natural sources

Sea salt, shellfish, carrots, beets, artichokes, dried beef.

SULFUR

Most people whose diet includes adequate protein are also getting enough sulfur.

Benefits

- promotes healthy *hair, skin, nails*
- applied in creams, helps treat various *skin problems*
- maintains oxygen balance for proper *brain function*
- supports the *liver* in bile secretion
- helps combat *bacterial infections*

Natural sources

Beef, fish, eggs, dried beans, cabbage.

VANADIUM

Vanadium taken in synthetic form can easily be toxic. However, it is rarely needed as a supplement.

Benefits

- cuts down formation of *cholesterol* in blood vessels
- helps prevent *heart attack*

Natural source

Fish.

ZINC

Alcoholics, diabetics, and those who take large doses of vitamin B6 need to increase their zinc intake.

Those who take extra zinc should also take extra vitamin A.

Benefits

- prevents _prostate_ problems
- helps control _cholesterol_ deposits and so prevents _arteriosclerosis_
- contributes to the formation of _insulin_
- aids in _healing of wounds_, both internal and external
- promotes _growth_ and _mental alertness_
- restores sense of _taste_
- helps treat _infertility_
- eliminates _white spots on fingernails_
- may help regulate _menstrual periods_

Natural sources

Eggs, yeast, wheat germ, nonfat dry milk, ground mustard, pumpkin seeds.

WATER

Water is an often forgotten element essential to proper health. Most people would benefit by increasing their daily water intake.

Thirst is the body's way of telling us that more water is needed. Extra glasses of water taken regularly throughout the day (and not just when one feels thirsty) would help most people.

Drink plenty of water! An ideal amount would be to drink about one glass of liquid (water) every two hours. For dieters, drink a full glass of water before each meal.

Benefits

- helps *keep all systems functioning*
- regulates body *temperature*
- prevents *constipation*
- aids in *dieting* by depressing appetite before meals
- prevents *dehydration*
- helps the body combat *fever, disease,* and *infection* by ridding it of impurities
- prevents the formation of kidney stones
- keeps the digestive tract functioning properly

Natural sources

Drinking water, juices, fruits, vegetables, distilled water (It's the last pure water in the earth; fruits are 90 percent distilled water.)

VITAMINS AND MINERALS FROM HERBAL SOURCES

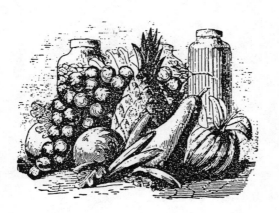

Many of the vitamins and minerals our bodies need can be obtained in natural forms—through herbs. Herbs are highly respected for their healing qualities. When a person takes them for their vitamin and mineral content as well, he's getting double benefit.

It may be that a major reason why herbs are so effective in body healing is the they are high in vitamins and minerals. We've included this section of the book for those who are concerned with natural health, and who would like to obtain their vitamins and minerals from the most natural source there is, the herbs that Mother Earth freely gives to us.

In this section we've listed some of the most popular herbs and their reported vitamin and mineral content. You can determine elsewhere in the book which vitamins and minerals your body needs. Then, if desired, you can get what you need from the herbs we've listed.

While you're at it, you may want to see how herbs use vitamins and minerals to do their work. Using this section, look up the herb you're interested in. See what vitamins and minerals it contains. Then move to the other sections of the book to see how those vitamins and minerals benefit the body. In that way you'll be able to better see how they assist the herb in its work as a healing agent. (Should you desire more information on herbs, we refer you to the companion volume of this work, *The Little Herb Encyclopedia*, also published by Thornwood Books.)

No one really knows *how* the body uses vitamins and minerals in its effort to keep healthy. We do know that they are essential for healthy living. We know that the body deteriorates and becomes sick if it doesn't have them—and can even die. And we know that they have certain medicinal properties that the body is able to utilize.

Herbs are much the same way. They have the ability to keep us healthy, even though oftentimes we don't know precisely how they work. But we do know they *do* work—and thousands of years of use has demonstrated that over and over again.

By combining our knowledge of the vitamin and mineral content of herbs with our understanding of many of the health benefits of those vitamins and minerals, we're able to come much closer to our goal of using the right things for the right reasons. As you use this section about the earth's natural healers you'll be able to approach that goal for yourself.

VITAMINS FROM HERBAL SOURCES

VITAMIN A

alfalfa, burdock, capsicum, dandelion, garlic, kelp, marshmallow, papaya, parsley, pokeweed, raspberry, red clover, safflower, watercress, and yellow dock.

VITAMIN B_1 (Thiamine)

capsicum, dandelion, fenugreek, kelp, parsley, safflower, raspberry.

VITAMIN B_2 (Riboflavin)

alfalfa, burdock, dandelion, fenugreek, kelp, safflower, watercress.

VITAMIN B_3 (Niacin)

alfalfa, burdock, dandelion, fenugreek, kelp, parsley, sage.

VITAMIN B_6 (Pyridoxine)

alfalfa.

VITAMIN B_{12} (Cyanocobalamin; Cobalt)

alfalfa, kelp.

VITAMIN C

alfalfa, burdock, boneset, catnip, capsicum, chickweed, dandelion, garlic, hawthorne, horseradish, kelp, lobelia, parsley, plantain, pokeweed, papaya, rose hips, shepherd's purse, strawberry, watercress, yellow dock.

VITAMIN D

alfalfa, watercress.

VITAMIN E

alfalfa, dandelion, kelp, raspberry, rose hips, watercress.

VITAMIN G

alfalfa, capsicum, dandelion, gotu kola, kelp.

VITAMIN K

alfalfa.

VITAMIN P (Rutin)

dandelion, rose hips.

VITAMIN T

plantain, alfalfa.

VITAMIN U

alfalfa.

MINERALS FROM HERBAL SOURCES

ALUMINUM

alfalfa.

CALCIUM

alfalfa, blue cohosh, chamomile, capsicum, dandelion, horsetail, Irish moss, kelp, mistletoe, nettle, parsley, plantain, pokeweed, pumpkin seeds, raspberry, rose hips, shepherd's purse, yellow dock, watercress.

CHLOROPHYLL

alfalfa.

CHLORINE

alfalfa, dandelion, kelp, parsley, raspberry.

COPPER

kelp, parsley, watercress.

FLUORINE

garlic, alfalfa.

IODINE

dulse, garlic, Irish moss, kelp, sarsaparilla, black walnut, dandelion.

IRON

alfalfa, burdock, blue cohosh, capsicum, dandelion, dulse, kelp, mullein, nettle, parsley, pokeweed, red beet, rhubarb, rose hips, strawberry leaves, yellow dock.

LITHIUM

kelp.

MAGNESIUM

alfalfa, blue cohosh, capsicum, dandelion, kelp, mistletoe, mullein, peppermint, primrose, raspberry, watercress, willow, wintergreen.

MANGANESE

kelp.

PHOSPHORUS

alfalfa, blue cohosh, caraway, capsicum, chickweed, dandelion, garlic, Irish moss, kelp, licorice, parsley, pokeweed, raspberry, rose hips, watercress, yellow dock.

POTASSIUM

alfalfa, blue cohosh, chamomile, comfrey, dulse, dandelion, eyebright, fennel, Irish moss, kelp, mistletoe, nettle, papaya, parsley, peppermint, plantain, raspberry, shepherd's purse, white oak bark, yarrow, wintergreen.

SELENIUM

alfalfa, kelp.

SILICON

alfalfa, blue cohosh, burdock, horsetail, kelp, nettle.

SODIUM

alfalfa, dandelion, dulse, fennel, irish moss, kelp, mistletoe, parsley, shepherd's purse.

SULFUR

alfalfa, burdock, capsicum, eyebright, fennel, garlic, Irish moss, kelp, mullein, nettle, parsley, plantain, raspberry, sage, shepherd's purse, thyme.

ZINC

kelp, marshmallow, licorice, ginseng, ho shou wu, damiana.

TRACE MINERALS

alfalfa, kelp. (boron, brominem nickel, strontium, vanadium)

APPENDIX

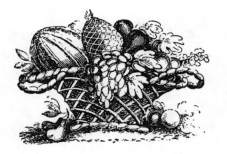

TABLE 1*

Some Nutrients Dependent on Each Other

*Supplied through the courtesy of the Nutrionics Literature Search, 624 N. Victory Blvd., Burbank, CA 91502 (213) 841-7200.

Nutrient	Complementary Nutrients	Anti-Vitamins	Bodily Functions Affected	Deficiency Symptoms
Vitamin A Fat soluble	B complex, choline, C, D, E, F, calcium, zinc	alcohol, coffee, cortisone, excessive iron, mineral oil, vitamin D deficiency	body tissue reparation and maintenance (resist infection). Visual purple production (necessary for night vision.	allergies, appetite loss, blemishes, dry hair, fatigue, itching burning eyes, loss of smell, night blindness, rough dry skin, sinus trouble, soft tooth enamel, susceptibility to infections
Vitamin B$_1$ Water soluble	B complex, B$_2$, folic acid, niacin, C, E, manganese, sulphur	alcohol, coffee, fever, raw clams, sugar (excess), stress, surgery, tobacco	appetite, blood building, carbohydrate metabolism, circulation, digestion (hydrocholoric acid production), energy, growth, learning capacity, muscle tone maintenance (intestines, stomach, heart)	appetite loss, digestive disturbances, fatigue, irritability, nervousness, numbness of hands & feet, pain & noise sensitivity, pains around heart, shortness of breath

TABLE 1 Continued

Nutrient	Complementary Nutrients	Anti-Vitamins	Bodily Functions Affected	Deficiency Symptoms
Vitamin B₂ Water soluble	B complex, B₆, niacin, C, phosphorus	alcohol, coffee, sugar (excess), tobacco	antibody & red blood cell formation, cell respiration, metabolism (carbohydrate, fat, protein)	cataracts, corner of mouth cracks & sores, dizziness, itching burning eyes, poor digestion, retarded growth, red sore tongue
Vitamin B₆ Water soluble	B complex, B₁, B₂, pantothenic acid, C, magnesium, potassium, linoleic acid, sodium	alcohol, birth control pills, coffee, radiation (exposure), tobacco	antibody formation, digestion (hydrochloric acid production), fat & protein utilization (weight control), maintains sodium potassium balance (nerves)	acne, anemia, arthritis, convulsions in babies, depression, dizziness, hair loss, irritability, learning disabilities, weakness
Vitamin B₁₂, Water soluble	B complex, B₆, choline, inositol, C, potassium, sodium	alcohol, coffee, laxatives, tobacco	appetite, blood cell formation, cell longevity, healthy nervous system, metabolism (carbohydrate, fat, protein)	general weakness, nervousness, pernicious anemia, walking and speaking difficulties

Nutrient	Complementary Nutrients	Anti-Vitamins	Bodily Functions Affected	Deficiency Symptoms
Biotin, B complex Water Soluble	B complex, B₁₂, folic acid, pantothenic acid, C, sulphur	alcohol, coffee, raw egg white (avidin)	cell growth, fatty acid production, metabolism (carbohydrate, fat, protein), vitamin B utilization	
Vitamin C Water Soluble	all vitamins & minerals, bioflavonoids, calcium, magnesium	antibiotics, aspirin, cortisone, high fever, stress, tobacco	bone & tooth formation, collagen production, digestion, iodine conservation, healing (burns & wounds), red blood cell formation (hemorrhaging prevention), shock & infection resistance (colds), vitamin protection (oxidation)	anemia, bleeding gums, capillary wall ruptures, bruise easily, dental cavities, low infection resistance (colds), nose bleeds, poor digestion
Vitamin D Fat Soluble	A, choline, C, F, calcium, phosphorus	mineral oil	calcium & phosphorus metabolism (bone formation), heart action, nervous system maintenance, normal blood clotting, skin respiration	burning sensation (mouth & throat), diarrhea, insomnia, myopia, nervousness, poor metabolism, softening bones & teeth

TABLE 1 Continued

Nutrient	Complementary Nutrients	Anti-Vitamins	Bodily Functions Affected	Deficiency Symptoms
Vitamin E Fat Soluble	A, B complex, B_1, inositol, C, F, manganese, selenium, phosphorus	birth control pills, chlorine, mineral oil, rancid fat & oil	aging retardation, anti-clotting factor, blood cholesterol reduction, blood flow to heart, capillary wall strengthening, fertility, male potency, lung protection (anti-pollution), muscle and nerve maintenance	dry, dull, or falling hair; enlarged prostate gland; gastrointestinal disease; heart disease; impotency; miscarriages; muscular wasting; sterility
Vitamin F Unsaturated fatty acids	A, C, D, E, phosphorus	radiation, x-rays	artery hardening prevention, blood coagulation, blood pressure normalizer, cholesterol destroyer, glandular activity, growth, vital organ respiration	acne, allergies, diarrhea, dry skin, dry brittle hair, eczema, gallstones, nail problems, underweight, varicose veins
Vitamin P Bioflavonoids	vitamin C	same as vitamin C	blood vessel wall maintenance, bruising minimization, cold & flu prevention, strong capillary maintenance	same as C (especially tendency to bleed & bruise easily)

Nutrient	Complementary Nutrients	Anti-Vitamins	Bodily Functions Affected	Deficiency Symptoms
Choline Water Soluble	A, B complex, B₁₂, folic acid, inositol, linoleic acid	alcohol, coffee, sugar (excessive)	lecithin formation, liver & gallbladder regulation, metabolism (fats, cholesterol), nerve transmission	bleeding stomach ulcers, growth problems, heart trouble, high blood pressure, impaired liver & kidney functions, intolerance to fats
Folic Acid Water Soluble	B complex, B₁₂, biotin, pantothenic acid, C	alcohol, coffee, stress, tobacco	appetite, body growth & reproduction, hydrochloric acid production, protein, metabolism, red blood cell formation	anemia, digestive disturbances, graying hair, growth problems
Inositol	B complex, B₁₂, B₂, C, Phosphorus	alcohol, coffee	artery hardening retardation, cholesterol reduction, hair growth, lecithin formation, metabolism (fat & cholesterol)	cholesterol (high), constipation, eczema, eye abnormalities, hair loss

TABLE 1 Continued

Nutrient	Complementary Nutrients	Anti-Vitamins	Bodily Functions Affected	Deficiency Symptoms
Niacin Water Soluble	B complex, B_1, B_2, C, phosphorus	alcohol, antibiotics, coffee, corn, sugar, starches (excessive)	circulation, cholesterol level reduction, growth hydrochloric acid production, metabolism (protein, fat, carbohydrate), sex hormone production	appetite loss, canker sores, depression, fatigue, halitosis, headaches, indigestion, insomnia, muscular weakness, nausea, nervous disorders, skin eruptions
Pantothenic Acid Water Soluble	B complex, B_6, B_{12}, biotin, folic acid, C	alcohol, coffee	antibody formation, carbohydrate, fat, protein conversion (energy), growth stimulation, vitamin utilization	diarrhea, duodenal ulcers, eczema, hypoglycemia, intestinal disorders, kidney trouble, loss of hair, muscle cramps, premature aging, respiratory infections, restlessness, nerve problems, sore feet, vomiting
PABA, Para Amino- benzoic Acid B complex	B complex, folic acid, C	alcohol, coffee, sulfa drugs	blood cell formation, graying hair (color restoration), intestinal bacteria activity, protein metabolism	constipation, depression, digestive disorders, fatigue, gray hair, headaches, irritability

Nutrient	Complementary Nutrients	Anti-Vitamins	Bodily Functions Affected	Deficiency Symptoms
Calcium	A, C, D, F, iron, magnesium, manganese, phosphorus	lack of exercise, stress (excessive)	bone & tooth formation, blood clotting, heart rhythm, nerve tranquilization, nerve transmission, muscle growth & contraction	heart palpitations, insomnia, muscle cramps, nervousness, arm & leg numbness, tooth decay
Chromium	none	none	blood sugar level, glucose metabolism (energy)	atherosclerosis, glucose intolerance in diabetics
Copper	cobalt, iron, zinc	zinc (high intakes)	bone formation, hair & skin color, healing processes of body, hemoglobin & red blood cell formation	general weakness, impaired respiration, skin sores
Iodine	none	none	energy production, metabolism (excess fat), physical & mental development	cold hands & feet, dry hair, irritability, nervousness, obesity

TABLE 1 Continued

Nutrient	Complementary Nutrients	Anti-Vitamins	Bodily Functions Affected	Deficiency Symptoms
Iron	B₁₂, folic acid, C, calcium, cobalt, copper, phosphorus	coffee, excess phosphorus, tea, zinc (excessive intake)	hemoglobin production, stress & disease resistance	breathing difficulties, brittle nails, iron deficiency anemia (pale skin, fatigue), constipation
Magnesium	B₆, C, D, calcium, phosphorus	none	acid alkaline balance, blood sugar metabolsim (energy), metabolism (calcium & vitamin C)	confusion, disorientation, easily aroused anger, nervousness, rapid pulse, tremors
Manganese	none	calcium, phosphorus (excessive intake)	enzyme activation, reproduction & growth, sex hormone production, tissue respiration, vitamin B₁ metabolism, vitamin E utilization	ataxia (muscle coordination failure), dizziness, ear noises, loss of hearing

Nutrient	Complementary Nutrients	Anti-Vitamins	Bodily Functions Affected	Deficiency Symptoms
Potassium	B6, sodium	alcohol, coffee, cortisone, diuretics, laxatives, salt (excess), sugar (excess), stress	heartbeat, rapid growth, muscle contraction, nerve tranquilization	acne, continuous thirst, dry skin, constipation, general weakness, insomnia, muscle damage, nervousness, slow irregular heartbeat, weak reflexes

Table 2
Recommended Optimum Personal Allowances (OPAs) for Vitamins

	Weight (±20 lbs.)	Height (±5")	Fat-Soluble Vitamins			Water-Soluble Vitamins (Essential)									Water-Soluble Vitamins (Contested)			
			Vitamin A (IU)	Vitamin D (IU)	Vitamin E (IU)	Vitamin C (mg)	Folic Acid (mcg)	Thiamin B1 (mg)	Riboflavin B2 (mg)	Niacin B3 (mg)	Vitamin B6 (mg)	Vitamin B12 (mcg)	Biotin (mcg)	Pantothenic Acid (mg)	Inositol (mg)	PABA (mg)	Pangamate (mg)	Bioflavonoids (mg)
MALES																		
Age: 19-35	147	69																
Lower limit			5,000	400	100	1,000	500	50	50	100	50	50	50	100	100	50	25	50
Upper limit			10,000	600	200	2,000	1,000	150	150	300	150	150	150	200	200	150	75	100
Age: 36-50	154	69																
Lower limit			5,000	400	200	1,000	500	100	100	100	100	100	100	100	100	100	25	50
Upper limit			10,000	600	400	3,000	1,000	150	150	300	200	150	150	200	200	150	75	100
Age: 51+	154	69																
Lower limit			10,000	400	400	2,000	500	100	100	200	100	100	100	100	100	100	25	50
Upper limit			15,000	600	600	4,000	1,000	200	200	400	200	200	200	300	300	200	50	100
FEMALES																		
Age: 19-35	128	65																
Lower limit			5,000	400	100	1,000	500	50	50	100	100	50	50	100	100	50	25	50
Upper limit			10,000	600	200	2,000	1,000	150	150	300	200	150	150	200	200	150	75	100
Age: 36-50	128	65																
Lower limit			7,000	400	100	1,000	500	100	100	100	200	100	100	100	100	100	25	50
Upper limit			12,000	600	300	3,000	1,000	150	150	300	300	150	150	200	200	150	75	100
Age: 51+	128	65																
Lower limit			10,000	600	400	2,000	500	100	100	200	100	100	100	100	100	100	25	50
Upper limit			15,000	800	600	4,000	1,000	200	200	400	200	200	200	300	300	200	50	100

NOTE: IU = International Units; mg = milligrams; mcg = micrograms.

BIBLOGRAPHY

Adams, Ruth. *The Complete Home Guide to All the Vitamins.* New York: Larchmont Books, 1972.

Adams, Ruth, and Murray, Frank. *Minerals: Kill or Cure.* New York: Larchmont Books, 1976.

Bieri, John G. "Fat-soluble vitamins in the eighth revision of the Recommended Dietary Allowances." *Journal of the American Dietetic Association* 64 (February 1974).

Borsaak, Henry. *Vitamins: What They Are and How They Can Benefit You.* New York: Pyramid Books, 1971.

Ebon, Martin. *Which Vitamins Do You Need?* New York: Bantam Books, 1974.

Goodhart, Robert S., and Shills, Maurice E. *Modern Nutrition in Health and Disease.* 5th ed. Philadelphia: Lea and Febiger, 1973.

Griffin, LaDean. *Please Doctor, I'd Rather Do It Myself . . . with Vitamins & Minerals.* Salt Lake City: Hawkes Publishing, Inc. 1979

Katz, Marcella. *Vitamins, Food, and Your Health.* Public Affairs Committee, 1971, 1975.

Martin, Marvin. *Great Vitamin Mystery.* Rosemont, IL: National Dairy Council, 1978.

Mindell, Earl. *Earl Mindell's Vitamin Bible.* New York: Rawson, Wade Publishers, Inc., 1980.

Null, Gary and Steve. *The Complete Book of Nutrition.* New York: Dell, 1972.

Rodale, J. I. *The Complete Book of Minerals for Health.* 4th ed. Emmaus, PA: Rodale Books, 1976.

Rosenberg, Harold, and Feldzaman, A. N. *Doctor's Book of Vitamin Therapy: Megavitamins for Health*. New York: Putnam's, 1974.

"Vitamin-Mineral Safety, Toxicity and Misuse." *Journal of the American Dietetic Association*, 1978.

Wade, Carlson. *Magic Minerals*. West Nyack, NY: Parker Publishing Co., 1967.

INDEX

A

A Vitamin 17, 18, 19, 20, 21, 22, 23, 24, 25, 26, 28, 29, 30, 31, 32, 33, 34, 35, 36, 43, 51, 52, 55, 57, 58, 79
Acne 17, 43, 59
Adrenal glands 17
Aging 17, 50, 58, 77
Air sickness 44, 48
Alcoholism 17, 44, 45,, 79
Alfalfa 61
Allergies 17, 56, 60, 76
Almonds 59
Amnesia 17
Anemia 17, 48, 49, 55, 56, 64, 71, 73, 75
Angina 17, 51
Antibiotics 47, 63
Antibodies 47, 48
Anxiety 44
Appetite 18, 49, 55
Apples 52, 74
Apricots 52, 55, 62
Arteriosclerosis 18, 46, 58, 70, 79
Arthritis 47, 76
Artichokes 77

Ascorbic acid 56
Asparagus 73
Aspirin 56
Asthma 18, 49, 51
Atherosclerosis 18, 53
Athlete's foot 23
Avocados 46, 55, 59

B

B_1 17, 18, 19, 22, 23, 24, 25, 26, 27, 28, 29, 30, 31, 33, 35, 36, 44, 46
B_2 17, 19, 22, 23, 24, 25, 27, 29, 30, 31, 32, 33, 34, 35, 45, 46
B_3 17, 18, 19, 20, 21, 22, 24, 25, 27, 28, 29, 30, 31, 32, 33, 34, 35, 46, 48
B_5 17, 18, 19, 21, 22, 23, 26, 29, 33, 34, 36, 47, 63
B_6 17, 18, 19, 21, 22, 24, 25, 26, 27, 28, 29, 30, 31, 32, 33, 34, 35, 36, 46, 48, 79
B_{12} 17, 18, 19, 20, 22, 23, 24, 27, 28, 29, 30, 33, 49, 55

B15 17, 18, 19, 21, 22, 23, 24, 25, 26, 27, 28, 29, 32, 34, 51
B17 20, 52
B Complex 17, 18, 19, 20, 21, 22, 23, 24, 25, 26, 27, 28, 29, 30, 31, 32, 33, 34, 35, 36
B vitamin factors 53, 54, 55
Back problems 56
Bad breath 18, 46
Balance 49
Baldness 18, 60
Bananas 48, 76
Beans 69, 71, 73, 75, 78
Bee stings 18
Beef 49, 77, 78
Beets 72, 75, 77
Beriberi 19, 44
Berries 57
Bioflavonoids 62
Biotin 53, 60
Birth control pills 44, 48, 55, 56, 58, 74
Birth defects 19
Blackberries 62
Bleeding (internal) 27, 56, 61
Blindness 19
Blood 19
Blood clots 19, 58
Blood clotting 19, 61
Blood disorders 47
Blood plasma 57
Blood pressure 19, 46, 54, 70, 76, 77
Boils 19, 43
Bones 19, 43, 56, 57, 69, 72, 76
Bones, broken 43

Bones, fractured 20, 56
Bran 44, 47, 48, 55, 63, 77
Brains (edible) 53
Brain functions 20, 46, 53, 78
Broccoli 57, 59, 77
Bronchitis 20
Brown rice 51
Bruises 20, 62
Burns 20, 56, 58, 63

C

C vitamin 17, 18, 19, 20, 21, 22, 23, 24, 25, 26, 27, 28, 29, 30, 31, 32, 33, 34, 35, 36, 55, 56, 57, 60, 62, 70, 71, 73, 74
C vitamin powder 23
Cabbage 53, 64, 72, 78
Caffeine 44, 53
Calcium 17, 18, 19, 20, 21, 23, 25, 26, 27, 28, 30, 31, 32, 33, 34, 35, 49, 57, 69, 72, 74, 76
Calcium deposits 74
Cancer 20, 52, 57, 77
Canker sores 20, 46, 55
Cantaloupe 48, 53, 55, 57
Carbon monoxide 56
Carbuncles 20, 43
Cardiovascular system 69, 74
Carrots 55, 77
Cauliflower 57
Cheese 45, 49, 69
Cherries 52, 62
Chicken pox 20

Iron 17, 21, 23, 24, 26, 28, 33, 56, 69, 71, 73, 75
Irritability 27, 49, 75

J

Joints 27
Juices 80

K

K vitamin 19, 20, 21, 25, 27, 28, 29, 31, 33, 35, 55, 61
Kelp 61, 70, 72, 77
Keratoconus 57
Kidney (edible) 45, 46, 47, 48, 49, 60, 63, 71, 73
Kidneys 27, 54, 76
Kidney stones 27, 48, 74, 80

L

Lactation 27, 31, 44, 48, 55, 57, 58, 72
Laetrile 52
Lecithin 20, 21, 28, 30, 32
Legs (cramps) 27
Lemon grass 43
Lemons 74
Lettuce 72
Lips 27, 45
Lima beans 53
Linseed oil 59
Liver 27, 43, 50, 51, 53, 54, 60, 78

Liver (edible) 44, 45, 46, 47, 48, 49, 53, 55, 60, 63, 71, 73
Lungs 27

M

Magnesium 21, 22, 24, 25, 27, 29, 30, 31, 34, 74
Manganese 17, 19, 22, 23, 27, 28, 29, 30, 32, 73, 75
Margarine 43
Measles 28
Meat (red) 46, 47, 48, 70, 71, 73, 76
Memory 49, 54, 75
Menopause 28, 58
Menstruation 28, 61, 69, 71, 73, 79
Mental alertness 72, 76, 79
Mental attitude 28, 44
Mental disorientation 28
Mental illness 29
Mental retardation 29
Metabolism 29
Migraine headaches 29, 46
Milk 43, 44, 45, 48, 49, 50, 57, 60, 69, 71, 79
Minerals 65-80
Mint leaves 76
Miscarriage (prevention) 29, 58, 62
Molasses 47, 48, 53
Molybdenum 17, 75
Mononucleosis 29
Morning sickness 29, 48
Motion sickness 29
Mouth 29, 45

Psoriasis 32, 43
Pumpkin seeds 51, 79
Pumpkins 55
Purpura 58
Pyorrhea 76
Pyridoxine 48

R

Radishes 72
Raisins 53
Red blood cells 48, 71
Reproductive system 32,
    43, 58, 75
Respiratory system 32, 43,
    58
Restlessness 32
Retinitis 58
Rheumatic fever 32, 58
Rheumatism 32
Riboflavin 45
Rice 44, 60
Rickets 33, 57, 69, 76
Rose hips 62
Rye flour 55

S

Safflower oil 59, 61
Salmon 57, 69
Sardines 57, 69
Scar tissue 58
Scurvy 33, 56
Sea salt 70, 77
Seafood 71, 72
Seasickness 44, 48
Seeds 54, 74, 76

Selenium 17, 20, 22, 28, 58,
    77
Sesame seeds 51, 63
Sex hormones 43, 46
Shellfish 70, 77
Shingles 33
Shock 33
Shrimp 71
Sinusitis 33
Skeletal system 58, 75
Skin 22, 33, 43, 45, 46, 48,
    55, 59, 63, 72, 73, 78
Skin disorders 33, 47, 58
Skin problems 43, 78
Smoking 44, 56
Sodium 22, 23, 29, 30, 34,
    77
Sore throat 34
Sores 34
Soybean oil 59, 61
Soybeans 48, 69
Spinach 59
Spinal disc 31, 34
Stress (mental & physical)
    34, 44, 45, 47, 56, 76
Sugar 44
Sulfa drugs 63
Sulfur 18, 20, 25, 26, 27, 28,
    30, 33, 34, 78
Sulfur cream 33
Sunburn 34, 63
Sunflower oil 59
Sunflower seeds 69, 76
Sunshine 57
Sunstroke 34, 77

T

T vitamin 17, 19, 25, 63

We're Interested!

Have you had good results using herbs? We're interested in hearing from you! Send your success stories to:

THORNWOOD BOOKS
Department D-12
1680 S. Main
Springville, Utah 84663

Health-Promoting Information

For a complete listing of our health-promoting information packed books, send your name and address to:

THORNWOOD BOOKS
1680 S. Main
Springville, Utah 84663

MORE BESTSELLERS
FROM THORNWOOD BOOKS!

☐ HERBAL AID by Edward Milo Millet ($2.95)
Which body systems are involved when you have a particular disease? *Herbal Aid* offers quick answers to your questions about herbs—nature's medicine.

☐ HERB SUCCESS STORIES—Volume 1 ($4.95)

Herbs work! Read these true stories submitted by people who have had terrific success using medicinal herbs.

☐ THE LITTLE HERB ENCYCLOPEDIA by Jack Ritchason ($3.95)
A companion to *The Little Vitamin and Mineral Encyclopedia*, this book answers the most commonly asked questions about using herbs to prevent or eliminate disease.

☐ GARLIC AT A GLANCE by Terry Tucker Francis ($1.00)
Garlic has been used for centuries to promote good health; find out why in this new book. Recipes for home remedies are included.

☐ A GUIDE TO NATURAL COSMETICS by Connie Krochmal ($5.95)
More than 550 all-natural recipes for making your own perfume, soap, lipstick, eye shadow, shaving cream, shampoo, and many other cosmetics.

☐ THE COMPLETE BOOK OF CAROB a cookbook by Frances Sheridan Goulart (Coming soon)
Here is the first book to give you more than a hundred recipes for using carob, nature's healthful chocolate alternative. Make beverages, cookies, cakes, brownies, pies, main dishes, and more!

☐ NATURAL HEALTH SECRETS OF THE STARS by Jill Williams (Coming soon)
Favorite home remedies, skin care and exercise tips, and healthful recipes are revealed by such favorite stars as Ron Howard, Charlene Tilton, Shirley Jones, Ricardo Montalban, Loni Anderson, Bob Barker, Vikki Carr, and 43 others.

Please send me the books I have checked. I have enclosed a check or money order for the amount of purchase, plus 15 % for postage and handling.

NAME _____

ADDRESS _____

CITY _____ STATE _____ ZIP _____

Please allow 3-4 weeks for delivery.